THE PICTURE BOOK OF
ANGELS

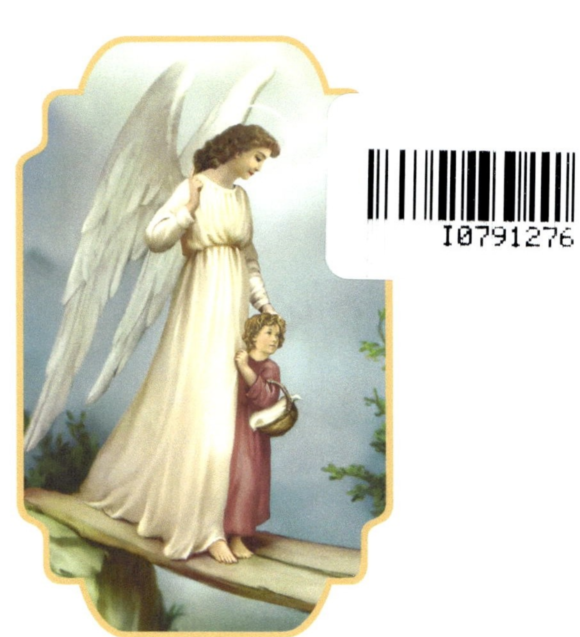

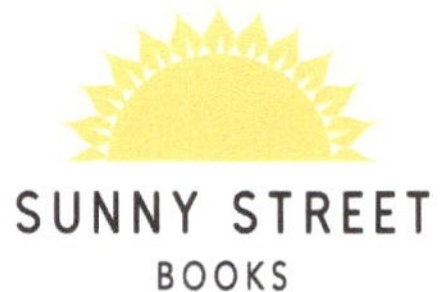

SUNNY STREET

BOOKS

$\mathcal{M}$usic is the

language spoken

by angels.

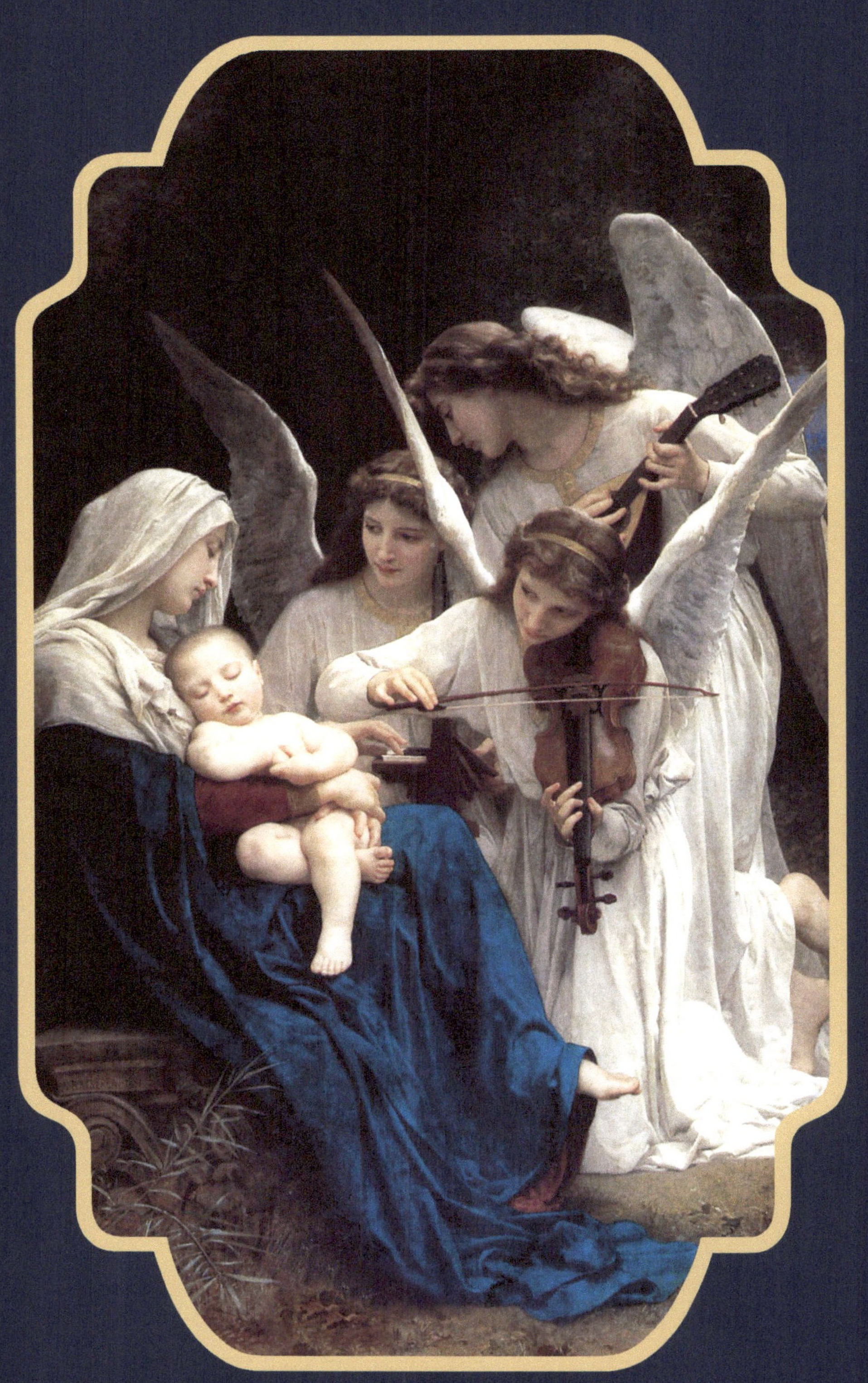

When life becomes
too much to bear,
remember your
angels are always
there.

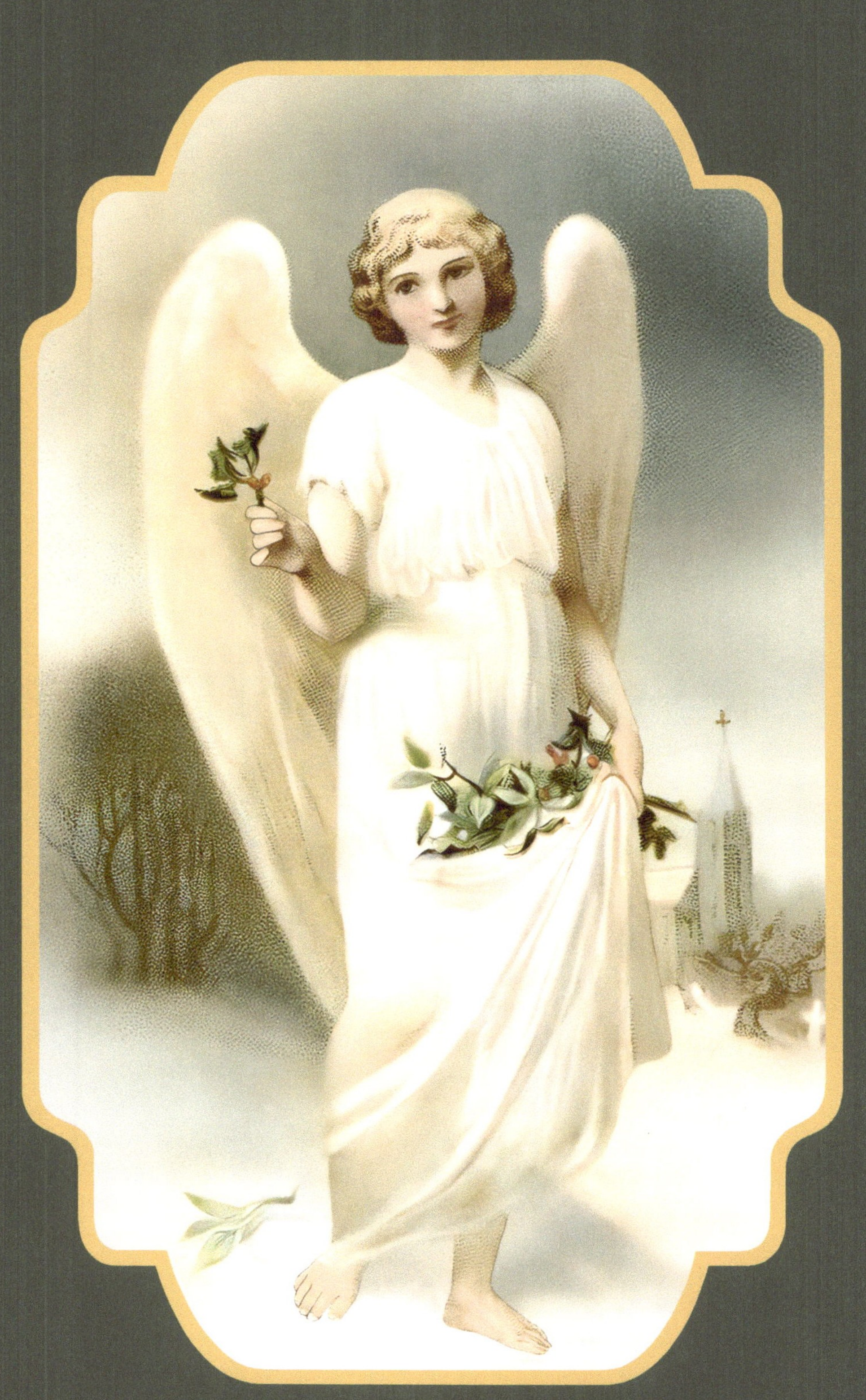

*I*f you have trouble hearing an angel's song, try listening with your heart.

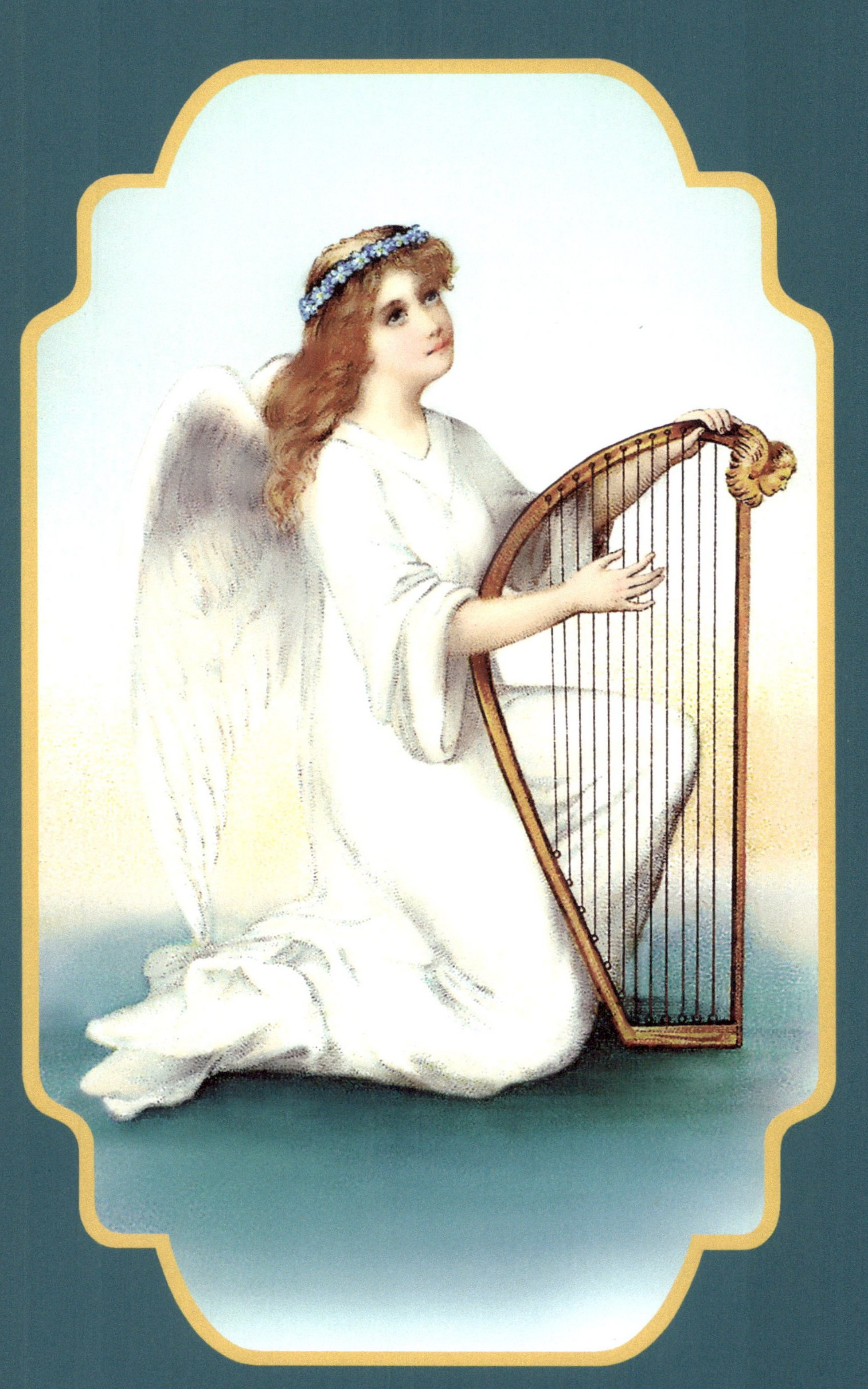

$\mathcal{B}$elievers, have
courage. The angels
are closer than you
think.

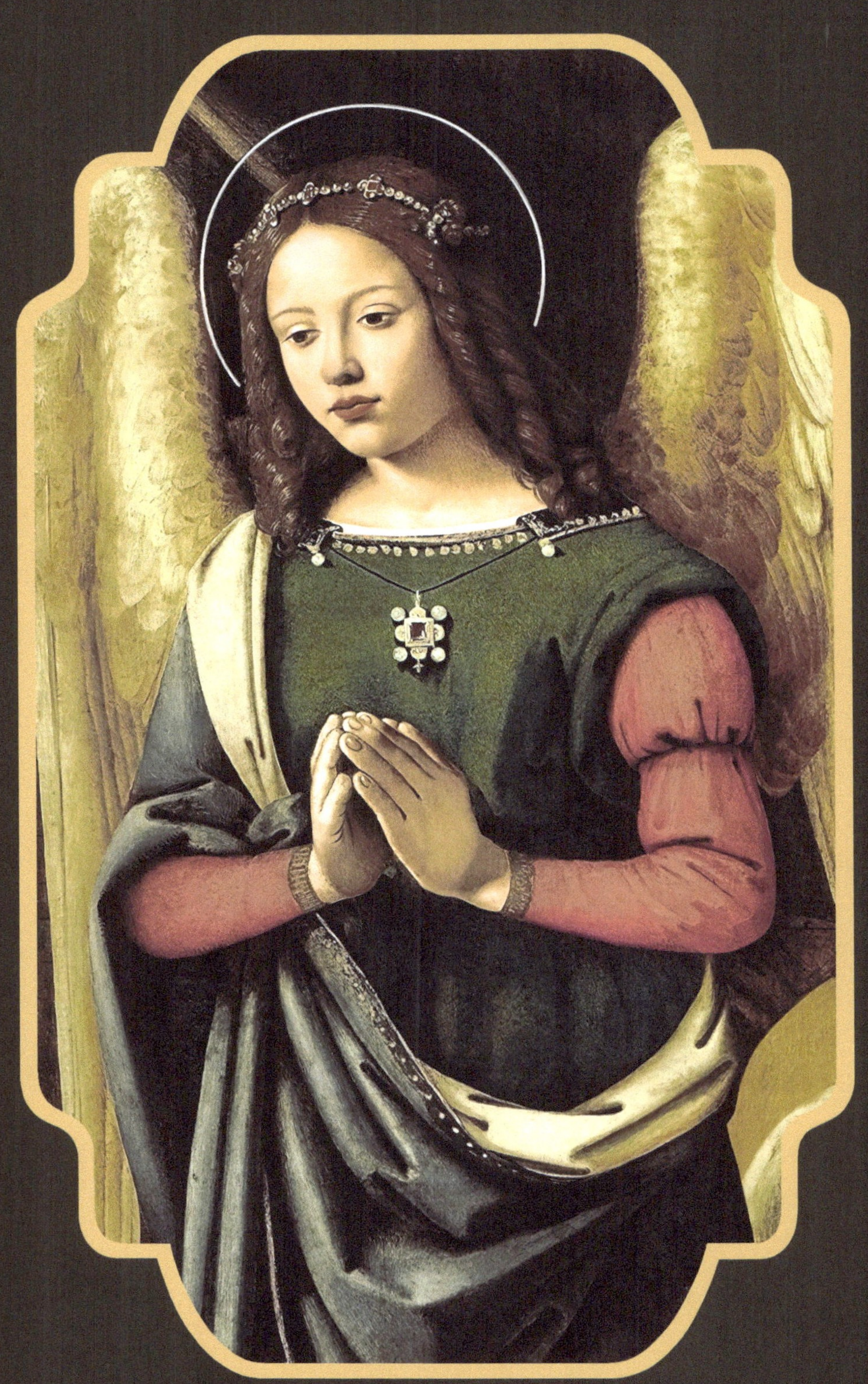

Wherever you go,

whatever you do,

may your guardian

angel watch over you.

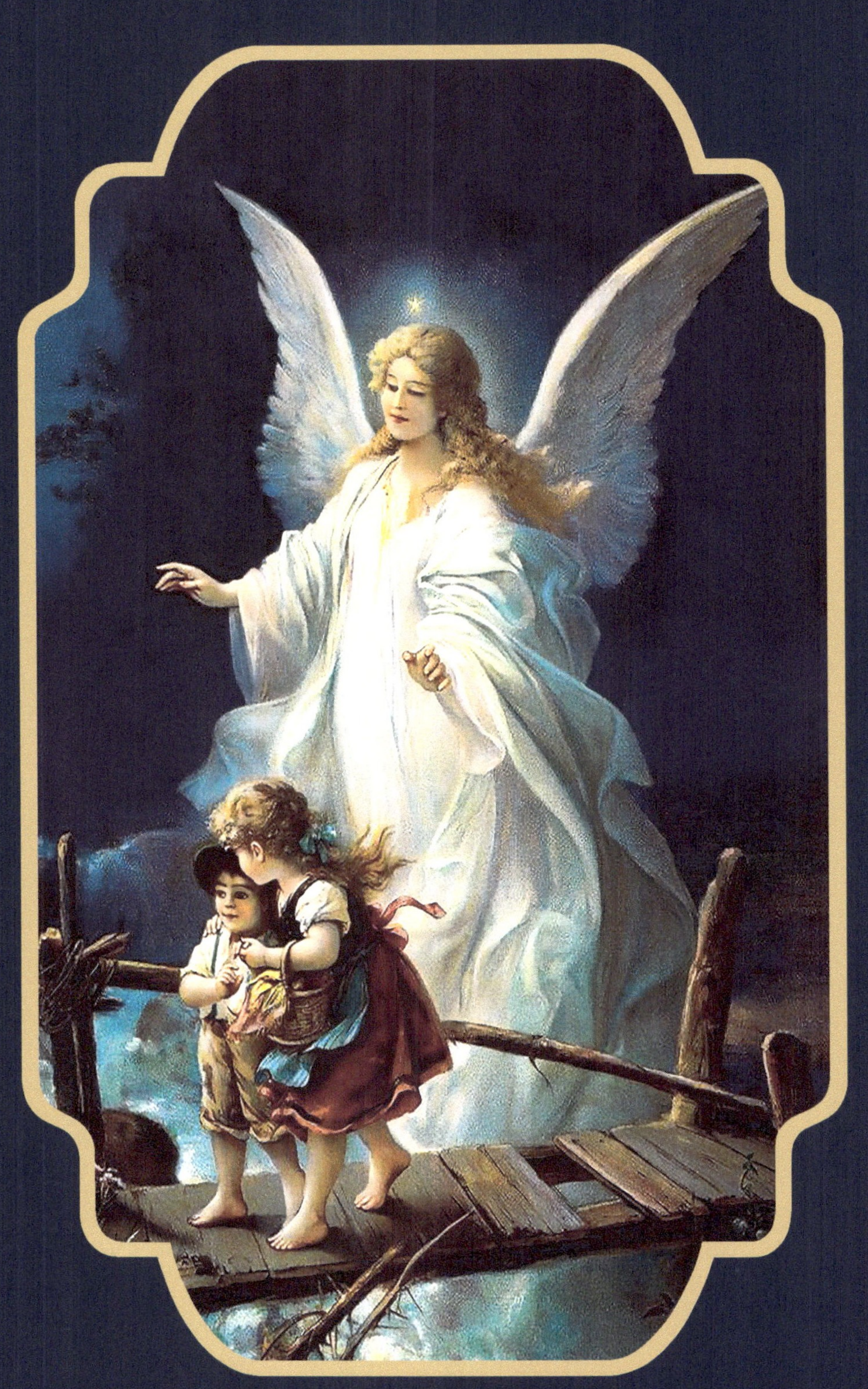

When you feel the presence of angels, you are feeling the love of God.

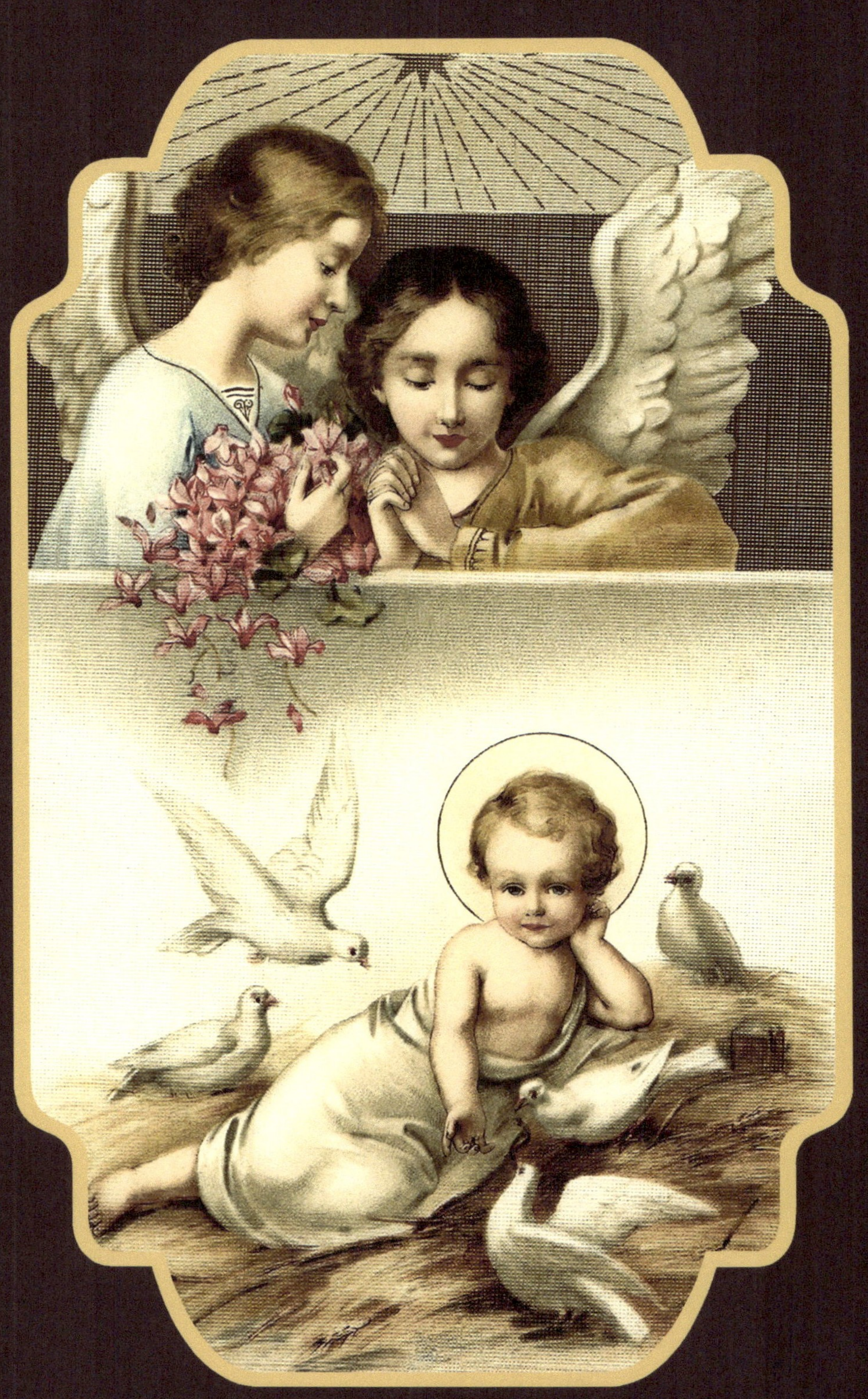

$\mathcal{E}$very time a bell rings, an angel gets their wings.

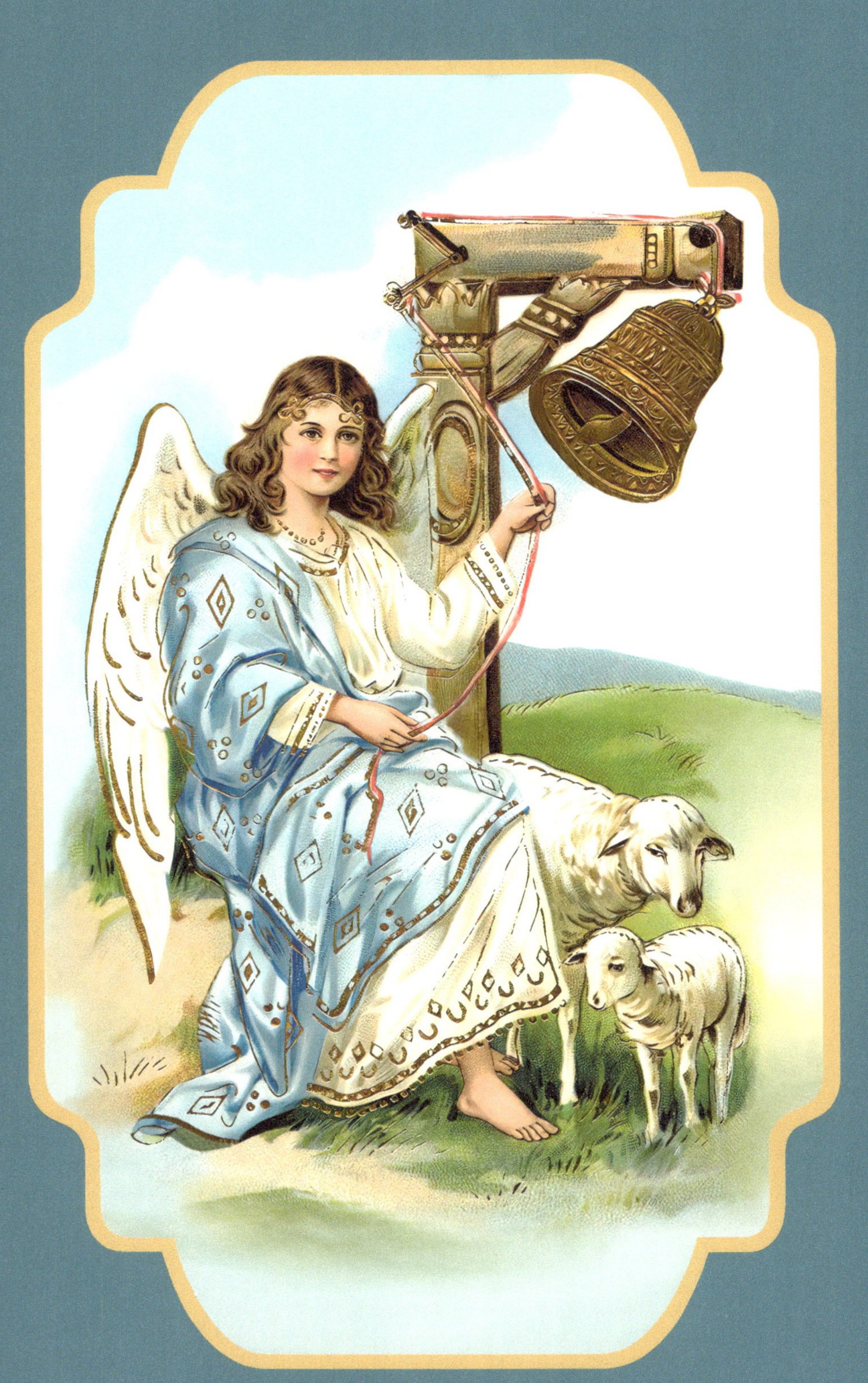

We are never so

lost that our angels

can't find us.

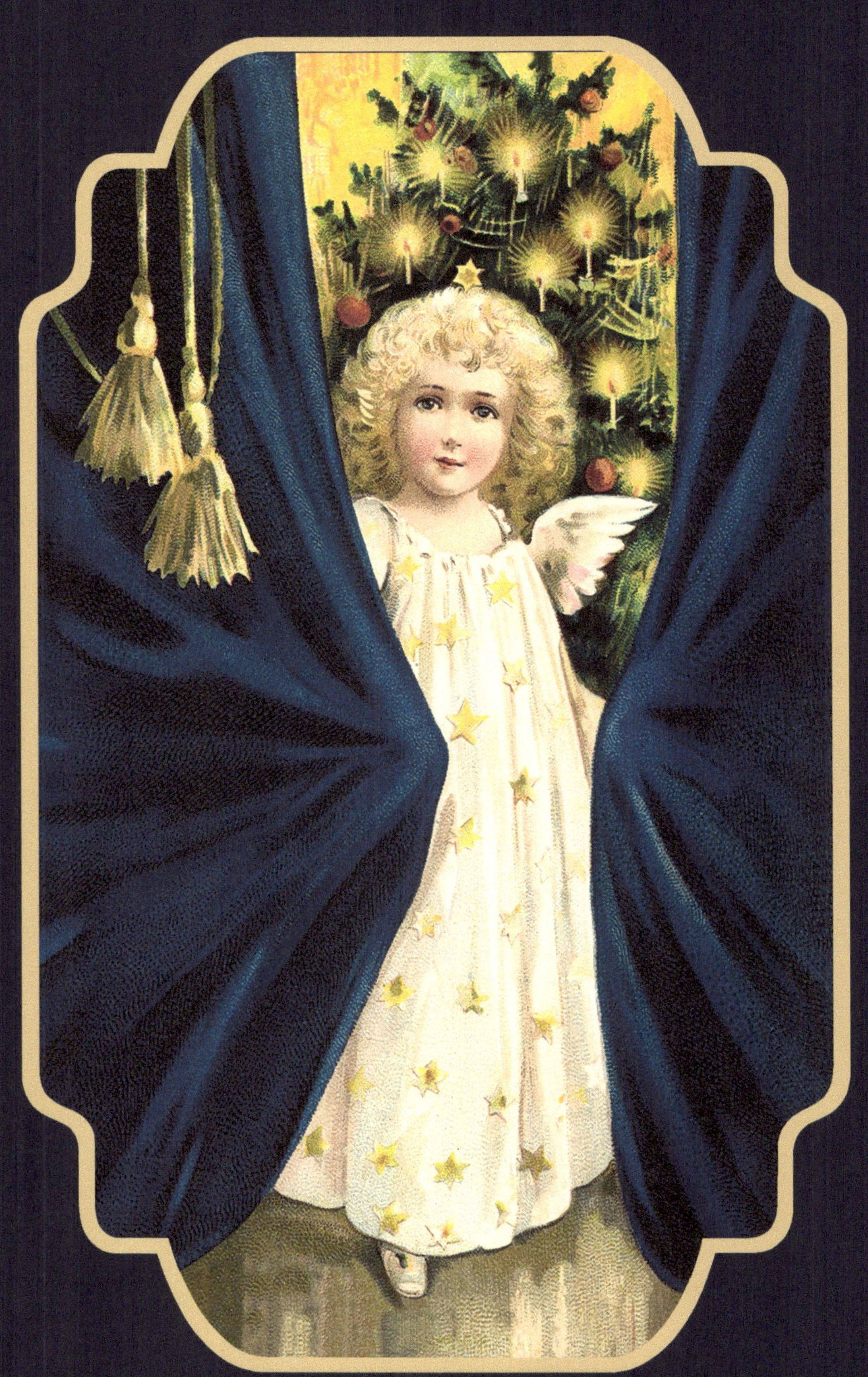

Angels guide us on

the path to happiness

and hope.

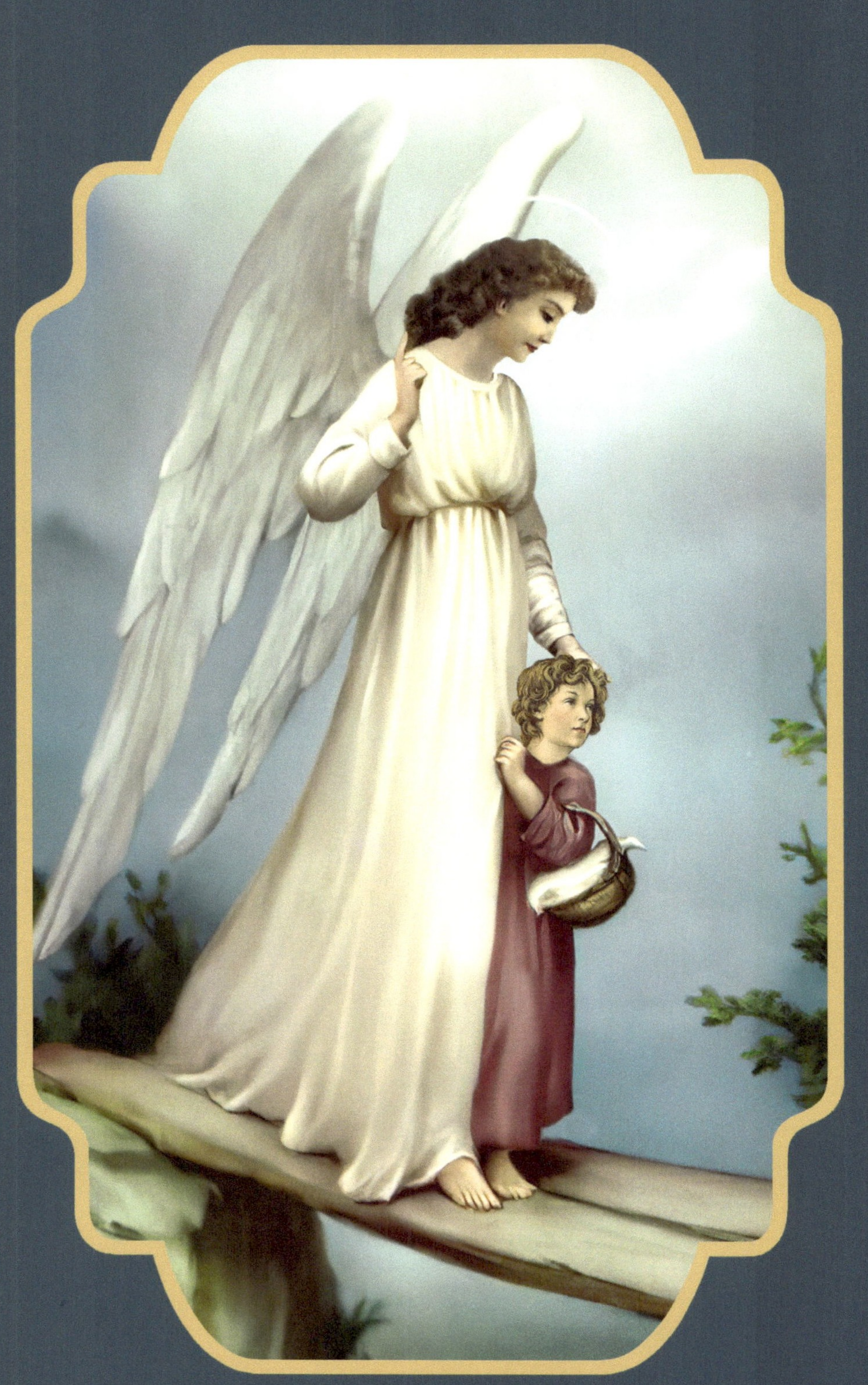

Guardian angels
sometimes fly beyond
our sight, but they are
always with us.

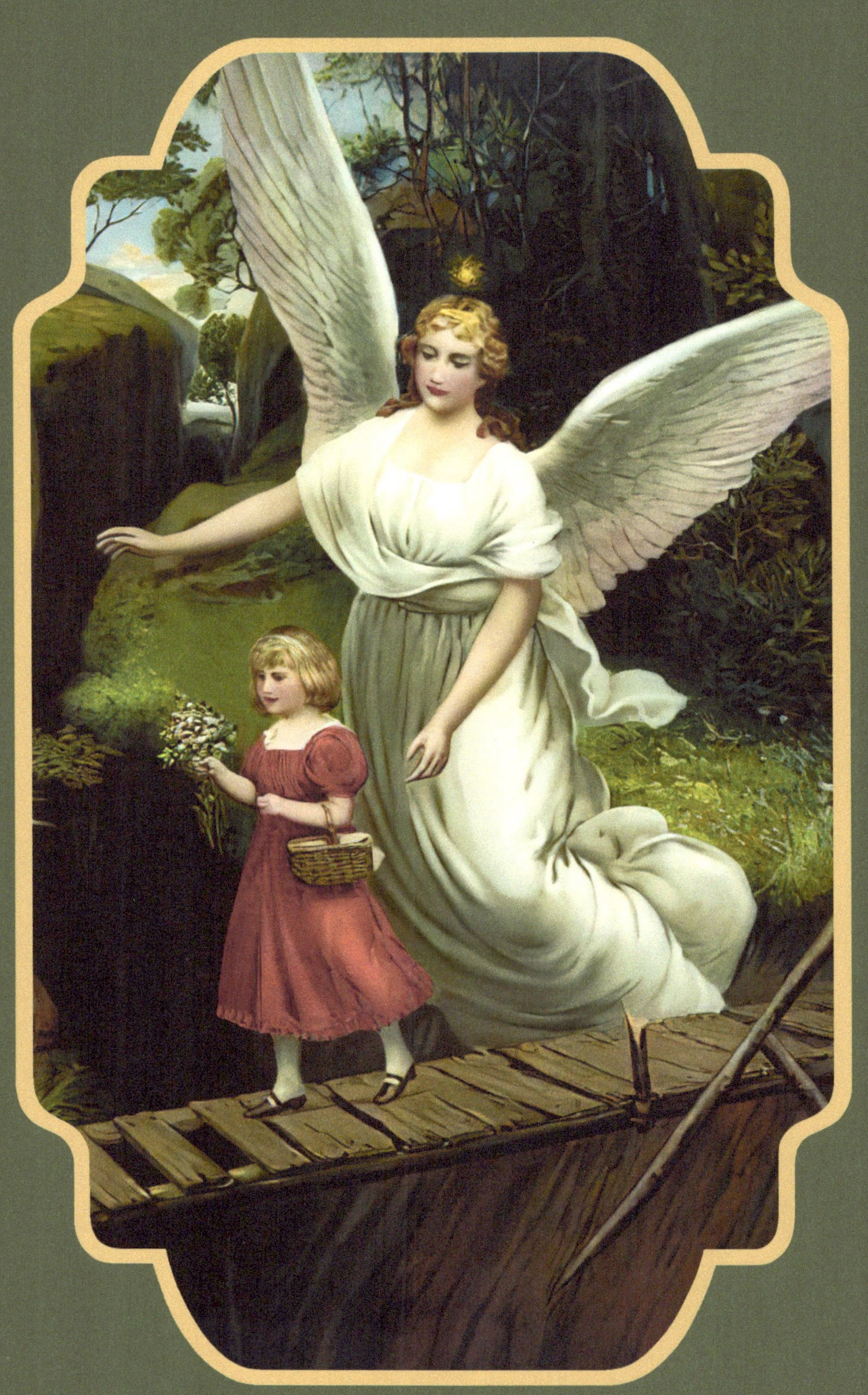

$\mathcal{M}$ay you travel

through life on the

wings of angels.

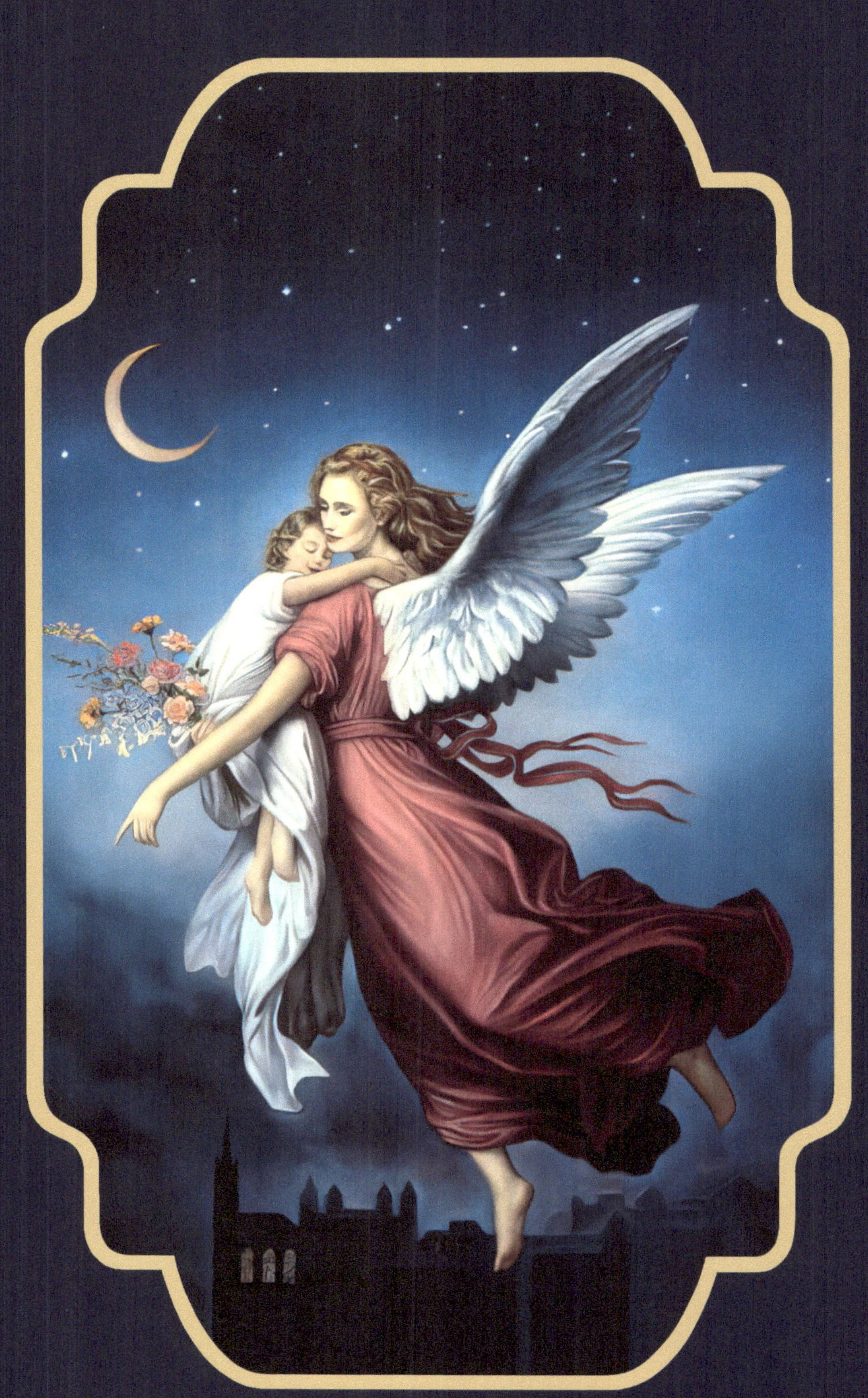

Our guardian angels
have endless patience.
They never, ever give
up on us.

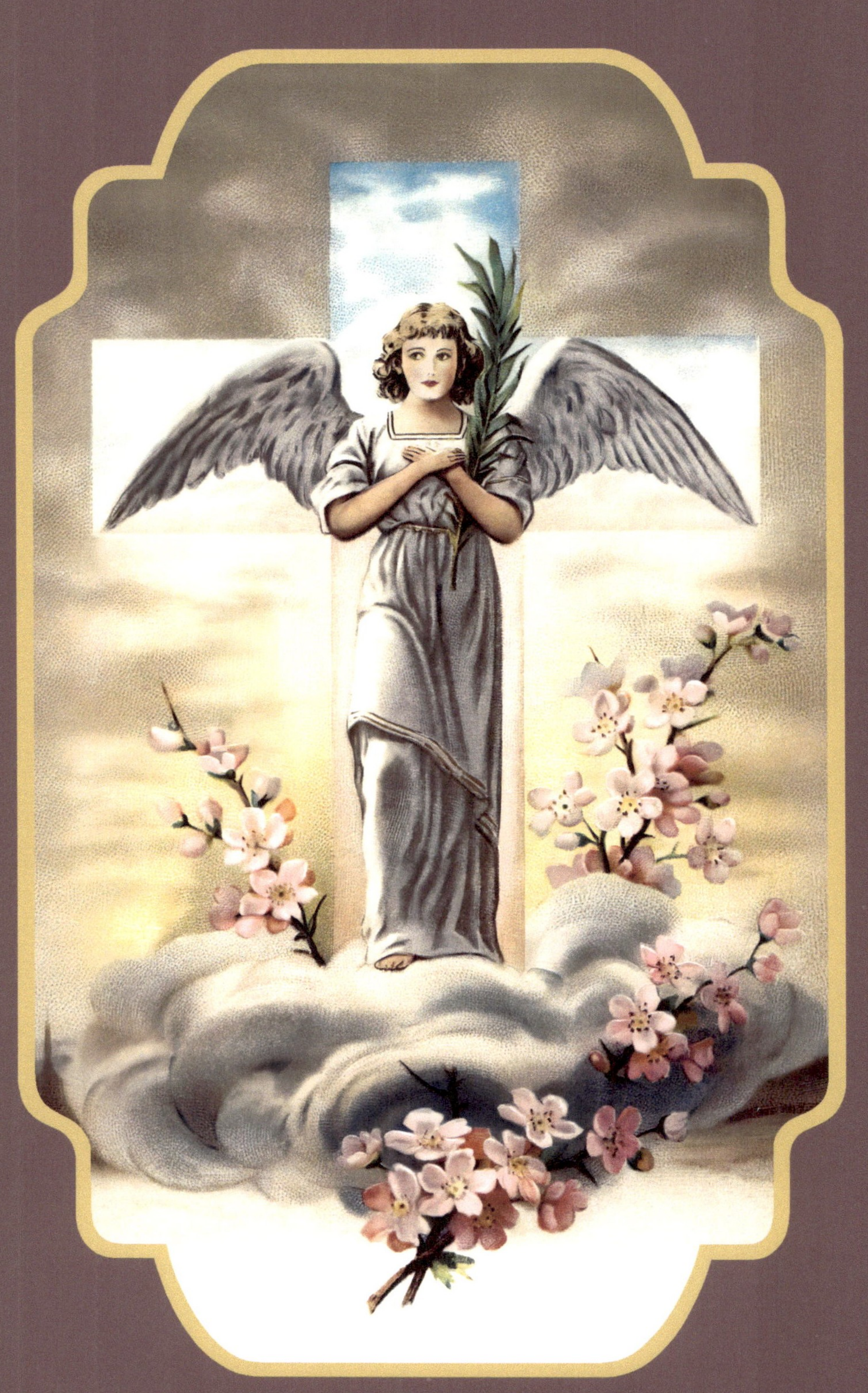

Ask your angel

to be near you, to

put a hand on your

shoulder, to give

you courage.

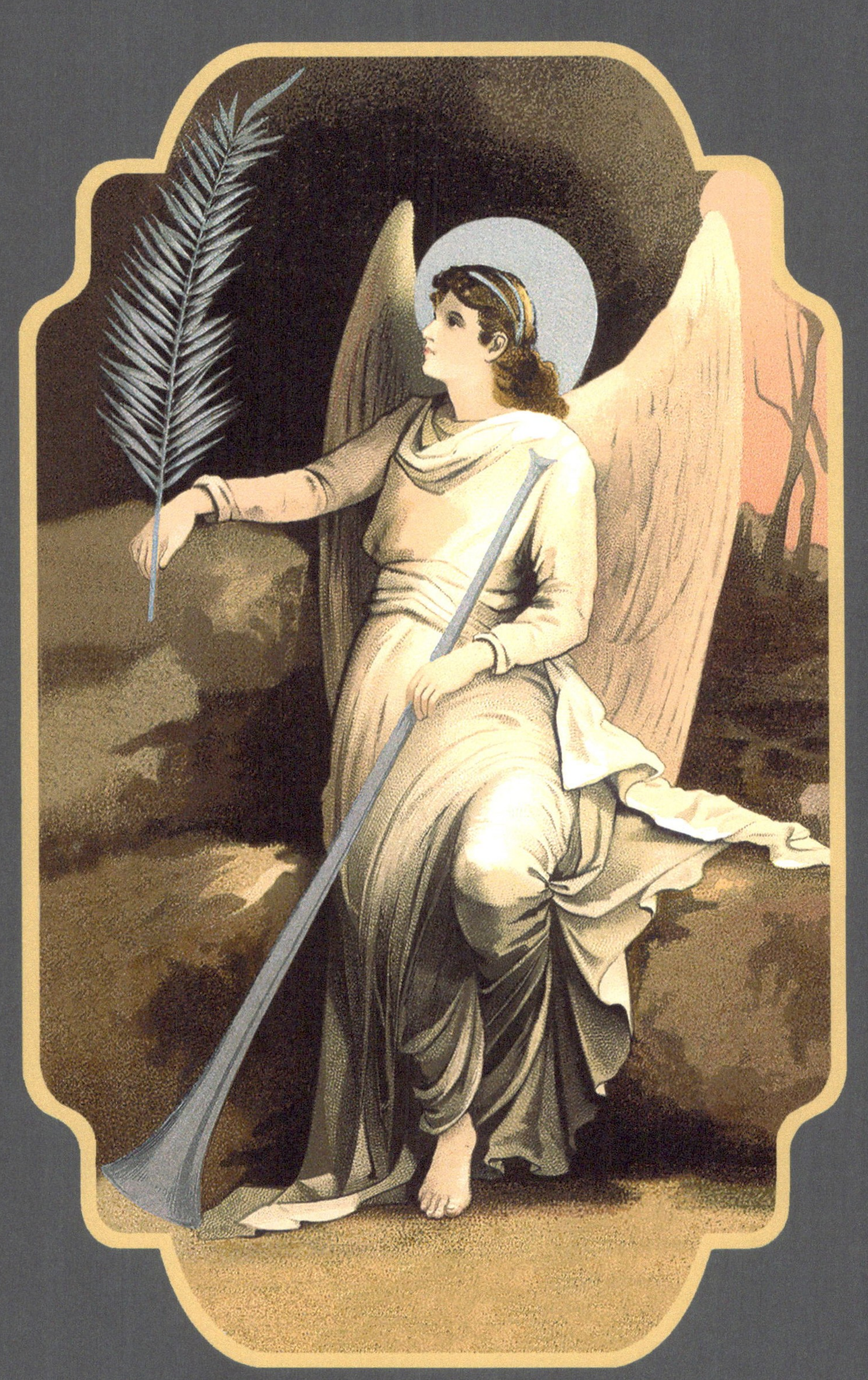

Guardian angel, pure
and bright, guard me
as I sleep tonight.

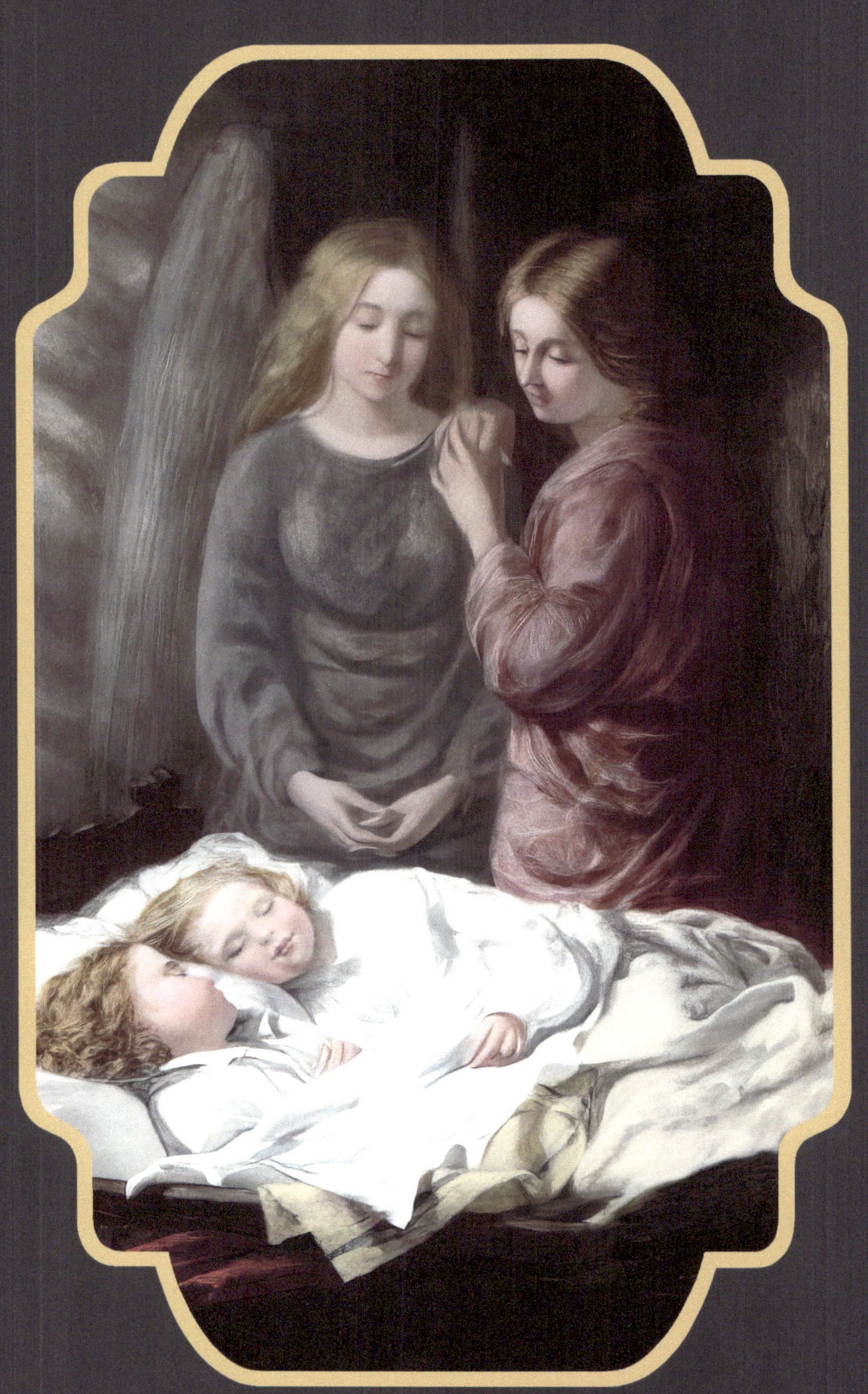

Snowflakes are angels

blowing their kisses

from heaven.

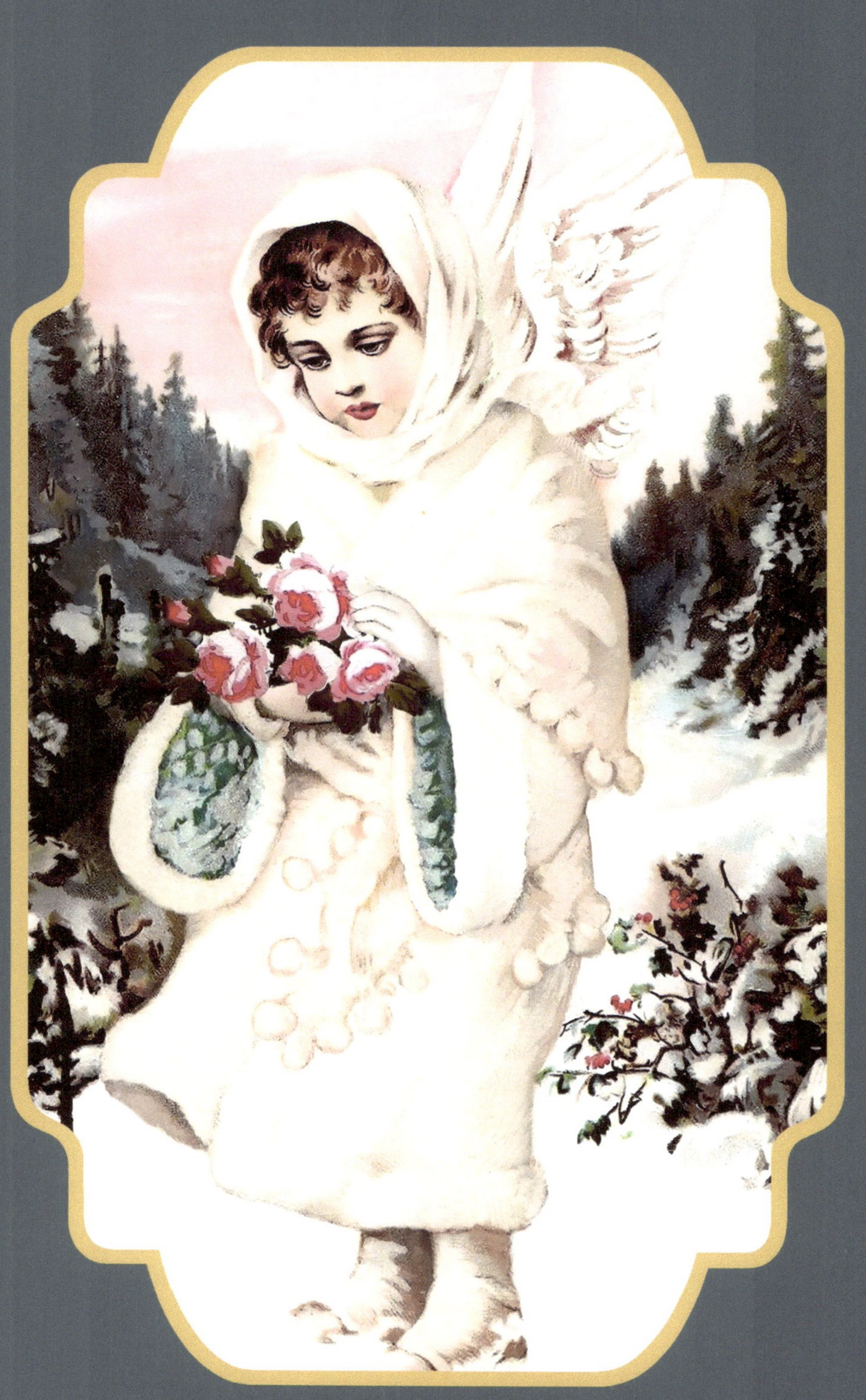

From the moment you take your first breath, angels are watching over you.

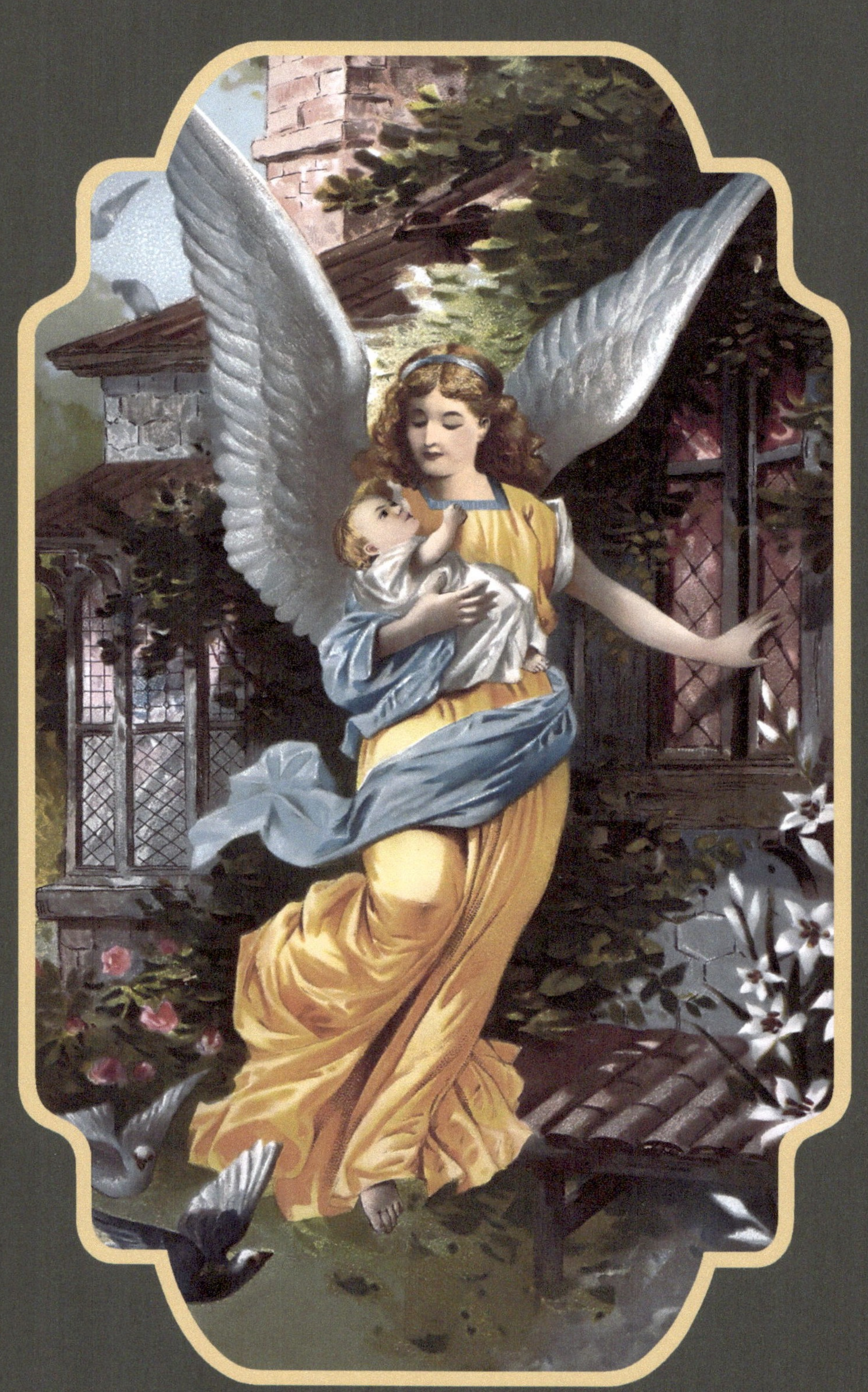

Angels descending,

bring from above,

echoes of mercy and

whispers of love.

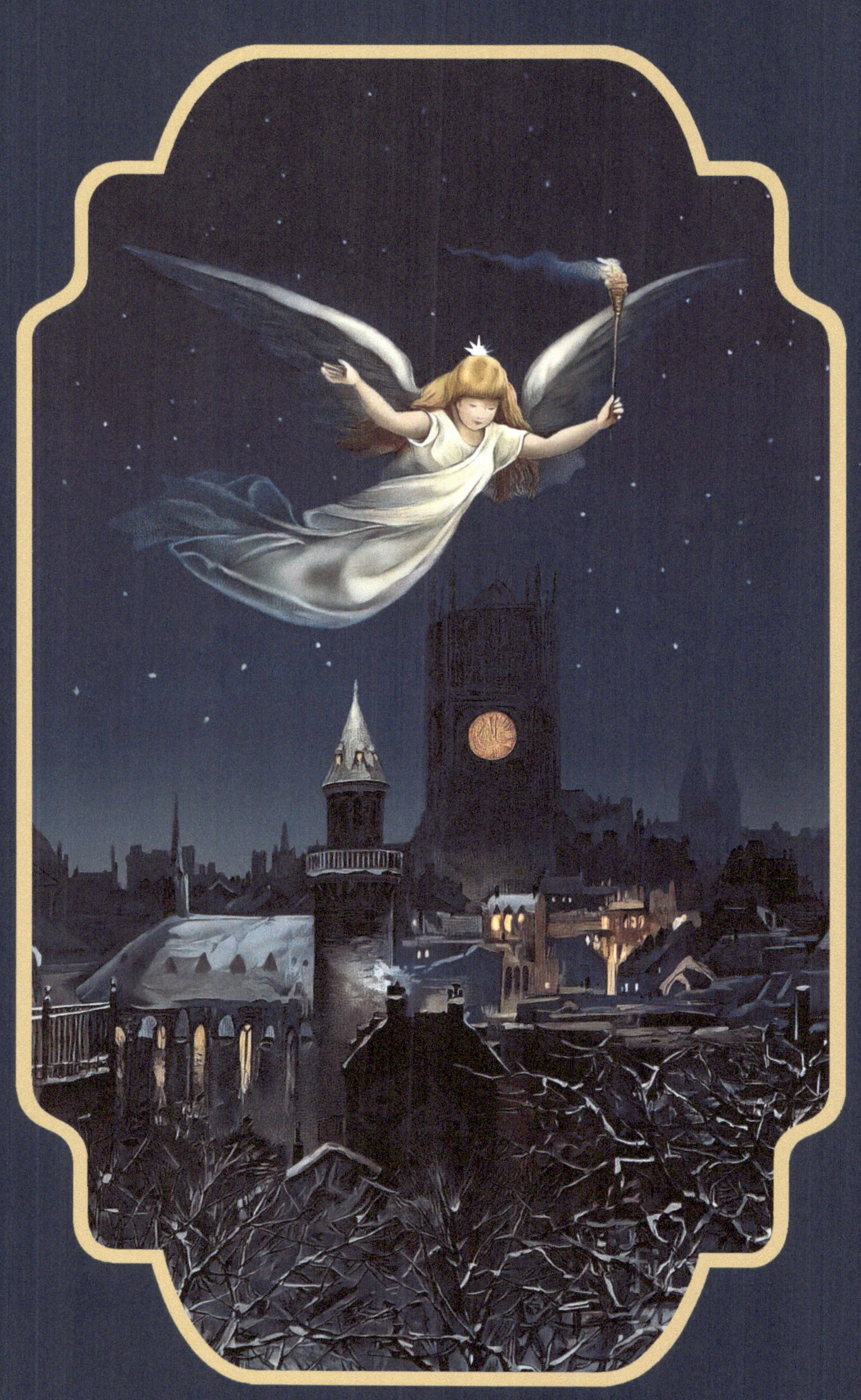

Angels are the guardians of hope and wonder, the keepers of magic and dreams.

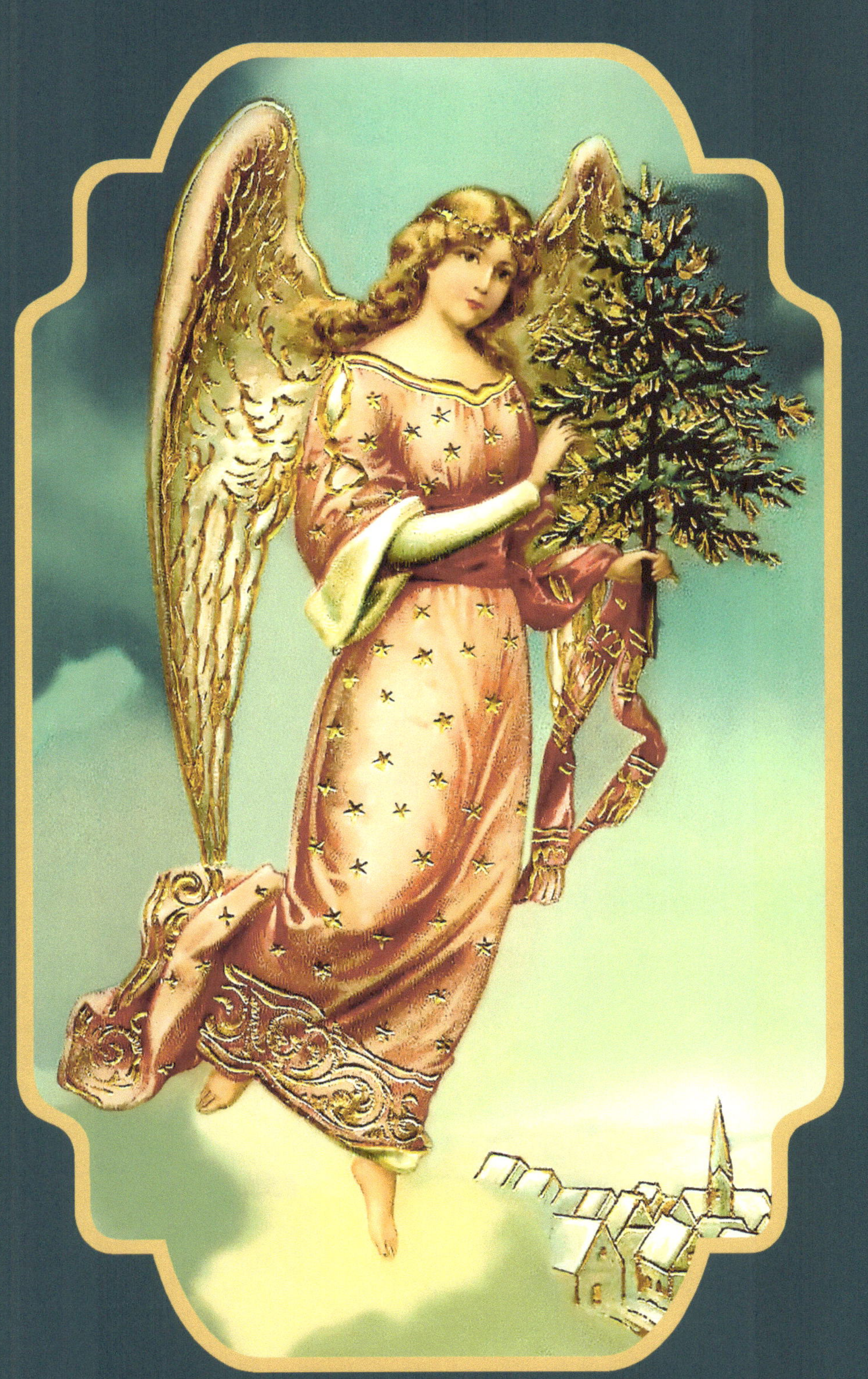

Angels are all
around us, all the
time, in the very air
we breathe.

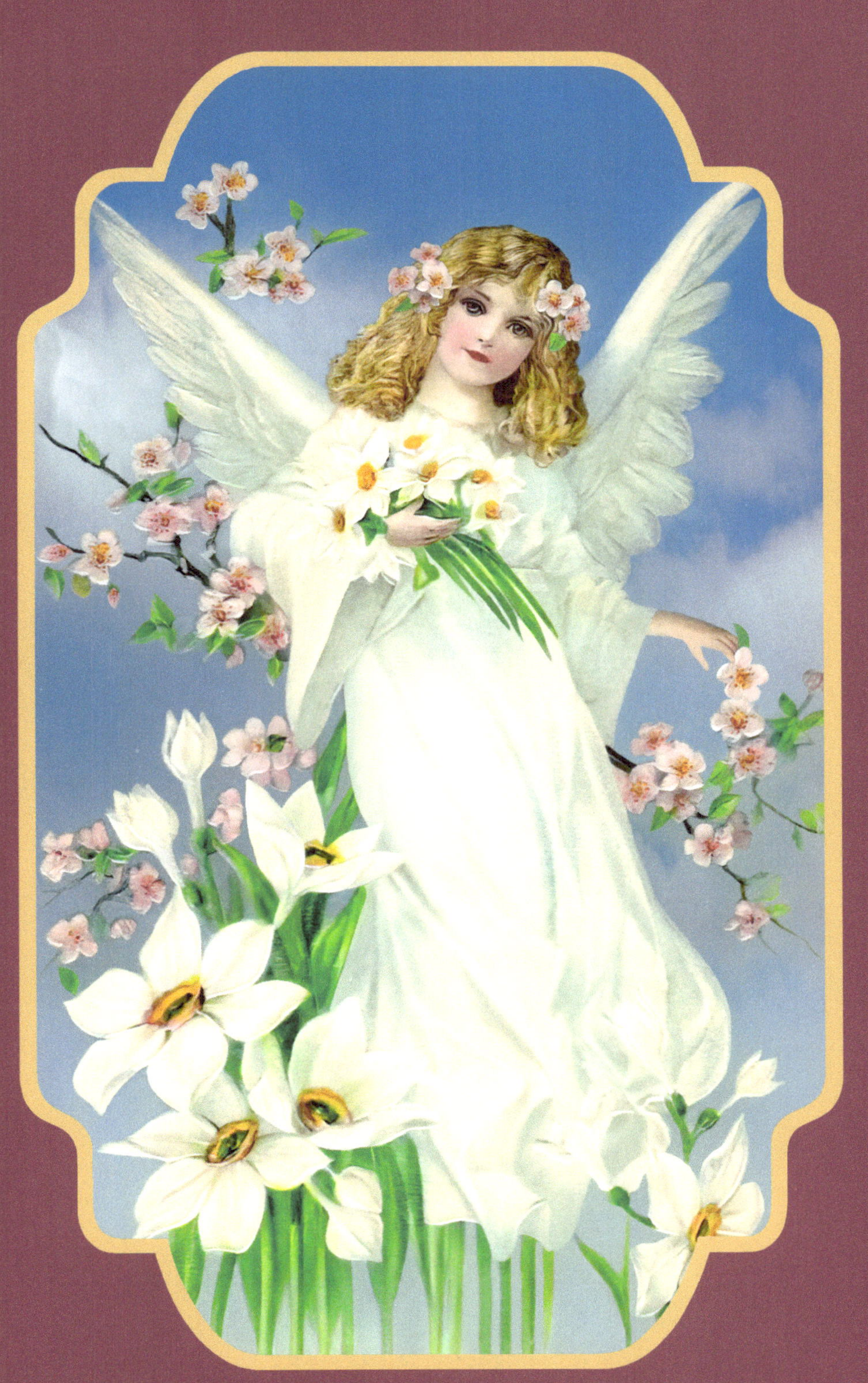

*H*appy is the

person who believes

in angels.

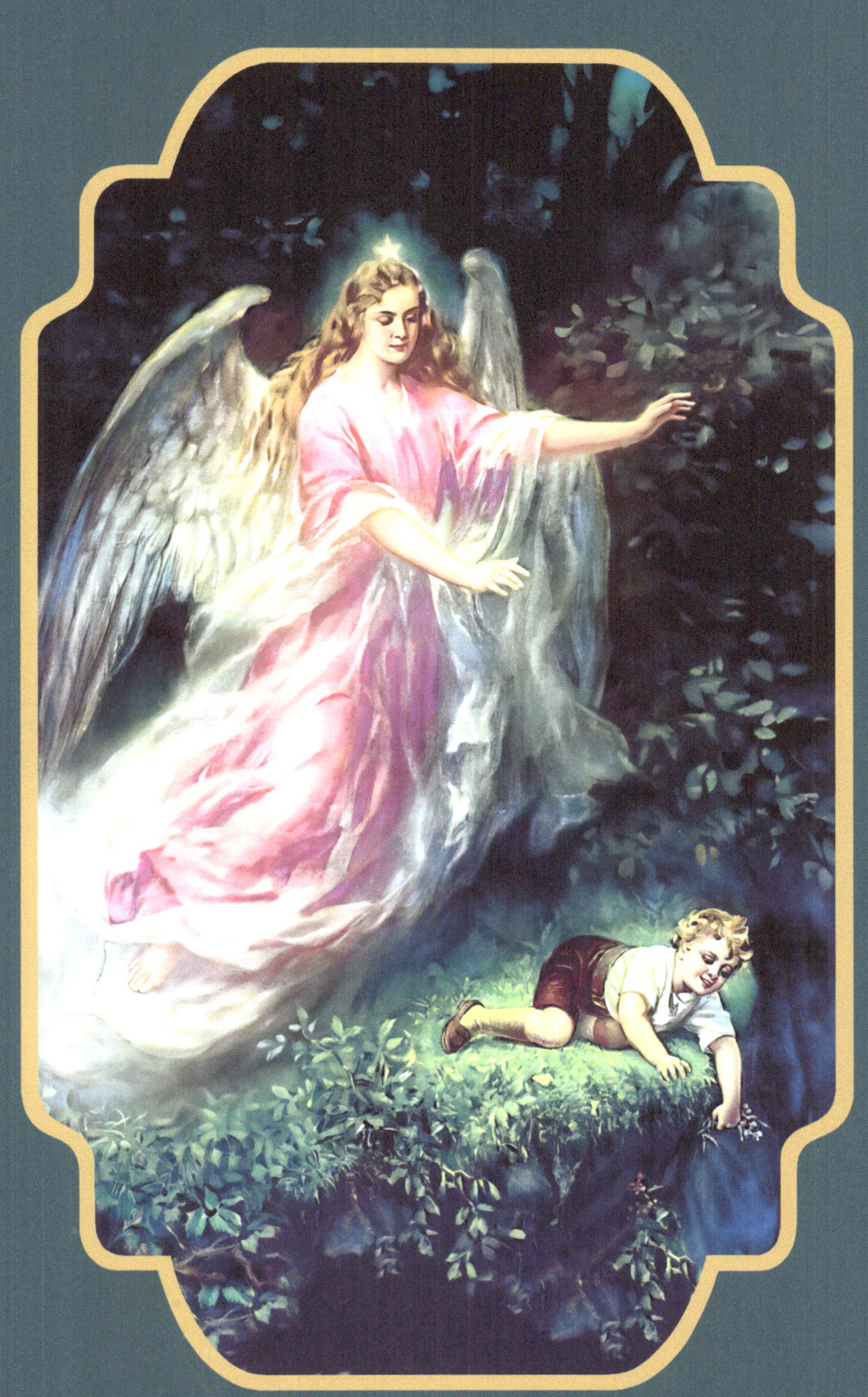

* 9 7 8 1 6 5 8 7 6 5 8 0 0 *